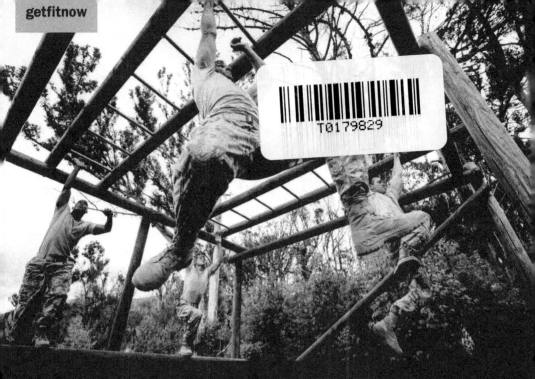

WARRIOR WORKOUTS

VOLUME 1

OVER 100 OF THE MOST CHALLENGING WORKOUTS EVER CREATED

INCLUDES: STRENGTH • CARDIO • ENDURANCE

STEWART SMITH, CSCS, USN (SEAL)

WARRIOR WORKOUTS VOLUME 1

Text Copyright © 2017 Stewart Smith

Library of Congress Cataloging-in-Publication Data is available.

ISBN: 978-1-57826-710-1

BOOK DESIGN BY CAROLYN KASPER

Printed in the United States

10 9

CONTENTS

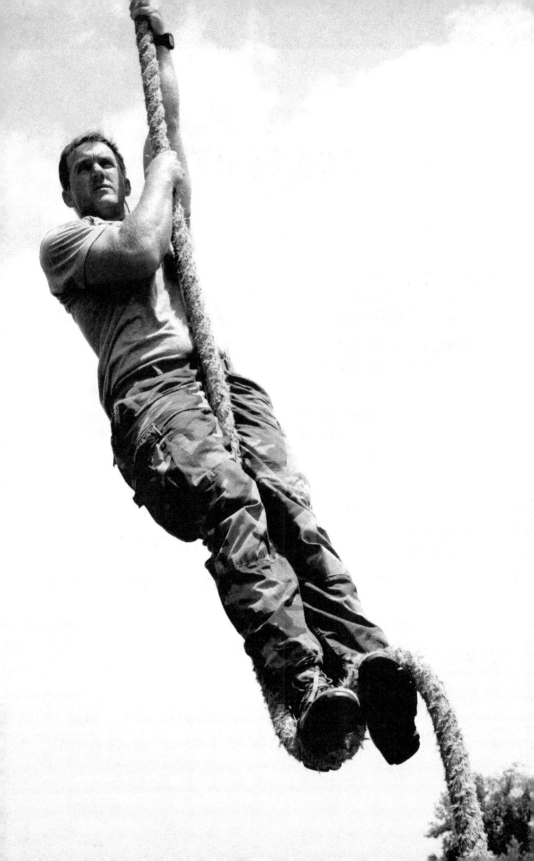

INTRODUCTION

A re you ready for results-driven workouts that will challenge you like no other exercise program available? Whether you are an everyday athlete, police officer, firefighter, or are in the military, *Warrior Workouts* is designed to push you to dig deep and find strength you never knew you had.

I am Stew Smith, creator of these workout arrangements. This book is jam-packed with workouts that have been thoroughly tested by myself and the Heroes of Tomorrow training groups for the past 15 years. Heroes of Tomorrow is a program designed to train young men and women for tactical professions like the military, police, firefighting, and more advanced SWAT and Special Operations programs. This training group yields successful special ops candidates (all branches/services), SWAT team members, FBI and local law enforcement, and firefighters every year.

In these workouts, you will see classics like PT pyramids arranged in new and different ways to give you methods to help make changes to break up the monotony of training. Doing the same workout week after week gets stale, after all, and eventually you'll need to make changes to your training plan to continue to see results. The 100 workouts in this book provide all the variety you need to keep you fit and in optimum physical condition.

These workouts are hardcore, but completely scaleable. Have fun and get creative with rearranging exercises and making changes to repetitions, distances, and events to fit your current fitness level and goals. No matter what your fitness goals, you will have *many* options to choose from with this book.

HOW TO USE THE WARRIOR WORKOUTS

The 100 stand-alone workouts in this book are some of my favorite workouts I have ever created. These are my top 100 individual workouts that focus mainly on calisthenics, running, swimming, rucking, and easy-to-use weights like dumbbells, kettlebells, sandbags, and backpacks. These are the most popular workouts that yield the most results for all of our top students seeking the toughest military, special ops, SWAT, and firefighting programs.

The workouts are organized into sections based on their category: upper body, upper body calisthenics and cardio, lower body calisthenics and cardio, full body calisthenics/resistance and cardio, and cardio and mobility workouts. Within each of these sections, you will find that the workouts are arranged in a somewhat random format, but each workout is titled with a description so that you can easily select the best workout for each day.

Some workouts are quick, while others require at least an hour to complete. Regardless, the goal is for you to do what you can on that day and arrange your workouts smartly. My advice on arranging the workouts into a complete week (5–6 days of training) would be as follows:

- Do your upper body workouts on Monday, Wednesday, and Friday. You can also add in cardio workouts after the upper body resistance workouts (cardio is often mixed into these particular workouts anyway).

- Add some leg days on the days in between (Tuesday, Thursday, and Saturday) or at least some form of cardio where you use your legs, such as running, biking, rucking, swimming (with fins), or rowing.

- With this type of volume—even in calisthenics—it is recommended to use the same muscle group *every other day* when it comes to resistance training to allow for maximum recovery and growth.

- Progress the cardio workouts logically to several days per week of running, biking, and swimming, but keep rucking at 2–3 times per week max for the purposes of these workouts.

The other option is to focus on full body workouts and do them every *other* day of the week, with rest or cardio days in between.

The rules are that simple!

NOTE: There are no exercise descriptions or pictures in this book. If you require a more detailed explanation of these standard exercises, all my other books have chapters devoted to exercise descriptions, with accompanying pictures. See the Resources section for a list of my other books. If there are any exercises you do not recognize, visit GetFitNow at getfitnow.com to find over 120 exercise videos, including some of the workouts in this book, to see the exercises in motion.

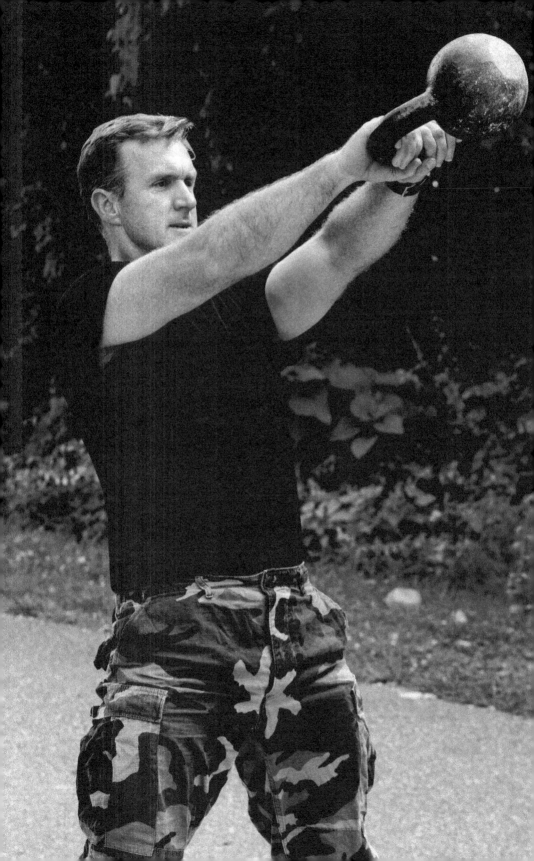

GENERAL TERMS

CSS Easy Pace: The Combat Swimmer Stroke (CSS) is the stroke many Special Ops programs require students to know, both with and without fins. When you see "easy pace", swim the CSS as a warm-up or a cool-down for the distance listed.

Dynamic Stretches: Increasing your flexibility should be the first goal before starting any fitness or athletic activity. Increased flexibility has been proven to aid in blood circulation, prevent injuries, increase speed, and improve range of motion. Dynamic stretches are the first step to warming up and preparing for your workouts. Take 5–10 minutes and get warmed up with the following leg movements prior to working out: jog or bike (5 minutes), Butt Kickers (1 minute), Frankenstein Walks (1 minute), Bounding in Place (1 minute), Side Steps (30 seconds in each direction), Leg Swings (1 minute), Calf/Shin Warm-Up (1 minute), Light Arm/ Shoulder/Chest Stretch, Light Thigh Stretch, Light Hamstring Stretch, Light ITB Roll, Shin Roll, and Hamstring Roll.

Easy Run: Running at a nice steady pace that is not too hard or too easy, but just above conversational pace. These types of runs are typical after hard resistance workouts or before a tough swim workout. Consider it an easy day of running for the distance listed when you see "easy run".

Free Hypox: Freestyle hypoxic swimming is also known as "skip breathing". Most people breathe every 3–4 strokes; however, to challenge yourself, try swimming 6–10 strokes per breath. To ensure safety, do *not* do this workout alone!

Light-Weight Shoulders: This refers to the following exercises: Lateral Raise, Thumbs Up Lateral Raise, Thumbs Up/Thumbs Down Lateral Raise, Front Raise, Cross-Overs, and Military Press. These should be done with no rest, using 3–5 pound dumbbells for 10 reps each.

Max Effort: Push yourself as hard and as long as you can, or as listed. For instance, usually this applies to 1–2 minute calisthenics tests, running timed runs, or swimming tests.

Physical Screening Tests (PST): Each branch of service has its own PT test. Take a pick of PT tests or challenge yourself and mix and match events to create your own PT test. For instance, the Navy SEAL, EOD, SWCC, Diver PST includes a 500 yard swim, Push-Ups test for 2 minutes, Sit-Ups test for 2 minutes, and a Pull-Up test (max reps) followed by a 1.5 mile timed run.

Pyramids: There are many types of pyramid workouts which you will see in this book. These workouts simply get harder on each set in repetition counts. For example, the Pull-Up, Push-Up, Sit-Up Pyramid is a classic, where you double the Push-Ups on each set and triple the Sit-Ups on each set in relation to your Pull-Ups numbers. So the first set looks like this: 1 Pull-Up, 2 Push-Ups, and 3 Sit-Ups. The second set looks like this: 2 Pull-Ups, 4 Push-Ups, and 6 Sit-Ups. If you go up to 10, 20, and 30 then back down the pyramid that equals 100 Pull-Ups, 200 Push-Ups, and 300 Sit-Ups. See right for an illustration:

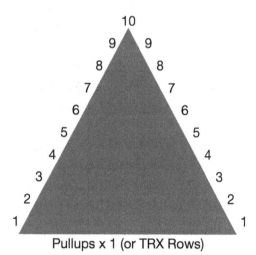

Pullups x 1 (or TRX Rows)

Pushups x 2 (or TRX atomic pushups)

Situps x 3 (or TRX Rollouts)

The other option is to focus on full body workouts and do them every *other* day of the week, with rest or cardio days in between.

The rules are that simple!

NOTE: There are no exercise descriptions or pictures in this book. If you require a more detailed explanation of these standard exercises, all my other books have chapters devoted to exercise descriptions, with accompanying pictures. See the Resources section for a list of my other books. If there are any exercises you do not recognize, visit GetFitNow at getfitnow.com to find over 120 exercise videos, including some of the workouts in this book, to see the exercises in motion.

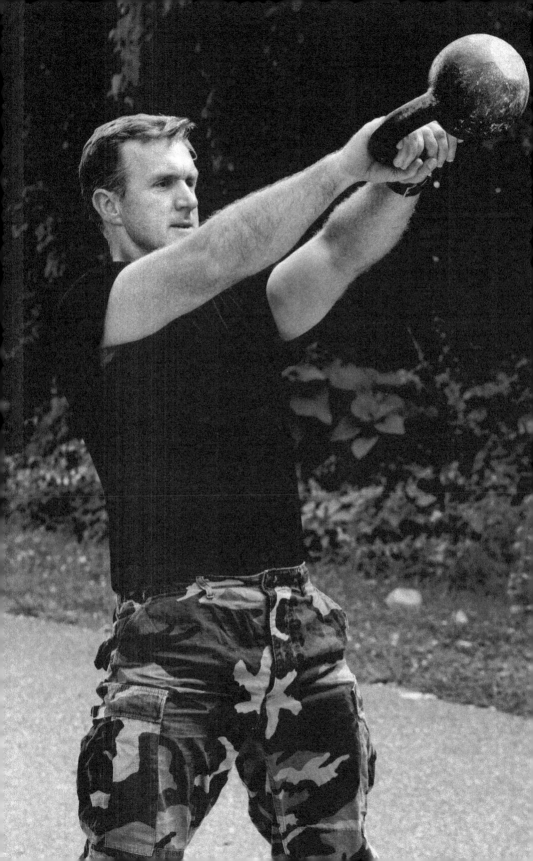

Revolutions Per Minute (RPM): This term applies to the bike pyramid to monitor your pedal speed. Typically, we keep the RPMs on a bike between 80–100 RPMs.

Sprint Free: Swim as fast as you can (sprint) using the freestyle stroke.

THE
WORKOUTS

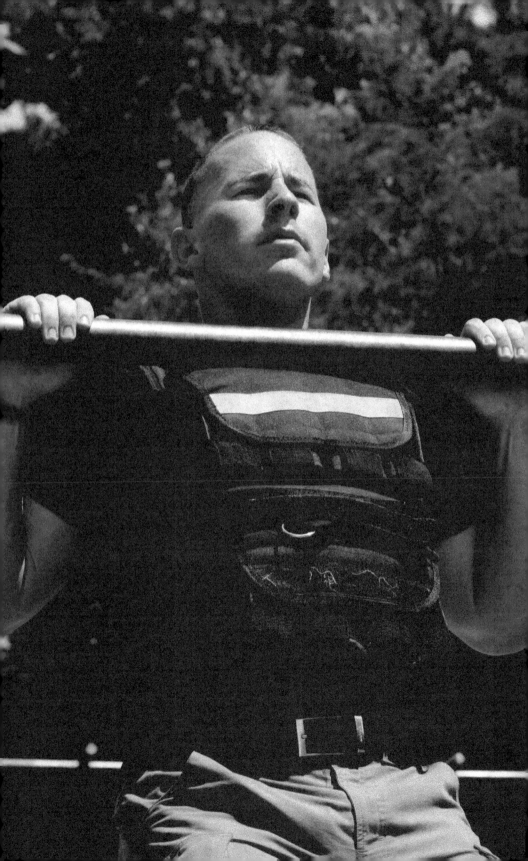

Upper Body

#1
PUSH-UP PT PYRAMID

(Good for building more balance into your training)

2-4-6-8-10 with 25 meter jogs/ dynamic stretches in between

Pull-Ups – max effort

Dips – max effort

Abs of choice (50) OR Plank Pose – 1 minute

Push-Ups Pyramid

12-14-16-18-20 with 25 meter runs in between

Pull-Ups max effort

Overhead Press (10–15) OR Hand
Stand Push-Ups (10–15)

Abs of choice (50) OR Plank Pose –
1 minute

Push-Ups Pyramid

22-24-26-28-30 with 25 meter runs
in between

Pull-Ups – max effort

Dips – max effort

Plank Pose – 1 minute

#2
BURPEE PYRAMID WARM-UP AND WORKOUT

Burpee Pyramid

1-2-3-4-5 with 25 meter jogs/dynamic
   stretches in between

Pull-Ups – max effort

Dips – max effort

Abs of choice (50) OR Plank Pose –
   1 minute

Burpee Pyramid

6-7-8-9-10 with 25 meter runs
   in between

Repeat 2 times

Pull-Ups – max effort

Dips (10–15)

Abs of choice (50)

Burpee Pyramid

11-12-13-14-15 with runs in between

Repeat 3 times

Pull-Ups – max effort

TRX Push-Ups OR Regular Push-Ups –
    max effort

Abs of choice (50) OR Plank Pose –
    1 minute

Burpee Pyramid

16-17-18-19-20 with runs in between

#3
FULL BODY PT WORKOUT

Warm-up: Run 5 minutes

Push-Up/Squat Pyramid 1–20 with 25 meter run in between sets: 1/1 Push-Up/Squat; run 25 meters; 2/2 Push-Ups/Squats; run 25 meters; 3/3 Push-Up/ Squat; run 25 meters; 4/4 Push-Up/Squat; run 25 meters...on every 5th set, do max Dips and Pull-Ups

Lightweight shoulders

Push/Pull/Leg/Core PT

Repeat 4 times

Pull-Ups – max

Push Press (10) or Hand Stand Push-Ups (10)

Squats (25) with no weight

Sit-Ups 1 minute OR Plank Pose – 1 minute

#4
SPECIAL USNA SUMMER SEMINAR WORKOUT

Run 1 mile/stretch

Repeat 10 times

Jumping Jacks (10)

Stretch 15 seconds (a muscle group each set)

Push-Ups: 5-10-15-20-25-30-35-40-45-50 = 275 Push-Ups

After each set of Push-Ups, stay in Push-Up or Plank Position for 15 seconds, then roll over and do:

Sit-Ups (20)

Flutterkicks, four count (25)

Then, stand up and do:

Squats (20)

Once done, do one extra set of 25 Push-Ups to get 300 total reps of Push-Ups

1 mile easy run

#5
ABS CIRCUIT

*(Great for a cool-down from a
    cardio workout with stretching
    mixed in)*

Repeat 2 times

Leg Levers (25)

Flutterkicks (25)

Plank Pose – 1 minute

Reverse Crunch (50)

Atomic Sit-Ups (25)

Regular Sit-Ups (50)

Left/Right Crunch (25 each)

Crunches (50)

Side Plank – 1 minute each side

Upper Body Calisthenics and Cardio: Running, Rucking, or Swimming

#6
DOUBLE NAVY SEAL PST

(Or, double the fitness test of your choice)

Swim – 500 yards

Push-Ups 2 minutes, Sit-Ups 2 minutes, Pull-Ups max effort

1.5 mile run

Rest 10 minutes

Repeat in reverse order

#7
CLASSIC PT PYRAMID WITH RUNNING BETWEEN SETS

Warm up with Pull-Up x 1; Push-Ups x 2; Sit-Ups x 3; Pyramid to 5 (dynamic stretches after each set for 25 meters). See below for details:

Set 1: 1 Pull-Up, 2 Push-Ups, 3 Sit-Ups, dynamic stretch, 25 meter run

Set 2: 2 Pull-Ups, 4 Push-Ups, 6 Sit-Ups, dynamic stretch, 25 meter run

Keep going using the x 1, x 2, x 3 system up the pyramid, stopping the dynamic stretches after the 5th set.

[Continued on next page]

Continue up the pyramid with sets 6, 7, 8, 9, 10

Repeat in reverse order – 10, 9, 8, 7, 6, 5, 4, 3, 2, 1

Run 1–2 miles for cool-down

#8
CLASSIC PT PYRAMID WARM-UP WITH RUNNING PT MIX

Warm-up with Pull-Up x 1; Push-Ups x 2; Sit-Ups x 3; Pyramid to 5 (perform dynamic stretches for 25 meters after each set)

Max Pull-Ups

Max Push-Ups 2 minutes

Max Sit-Ups 2 minutes

Run 1 mile

Max Pull-Ups

Max Push-Ups until you have to rest; stay in plank for extra 1 minute

Max Sit-Ups – 1 minute

[Continued on next page]

Run 1 mile

Max Pull-Ups

**Max Push-Ups until you have to rest;
    stay in plank for extra 1 minute**

Max Sit-Ups – 1 minute

Run 1 mile

#9
CLASSIC PT PYRAMID WITH 1-MILE RUNS

Warm up with Pull-Up x1; Push-Ups x 2; Sit-Ups x 3; Pyramid from 1–5 (perform dynamic stretches for 25 meters after each set)

Run 1 mile

Pull-Up x 1; Push-Ups x 2; Sit-Ups x 3; Pyramid from 6–10 (perform dynamic stretches for 25 meters after each set)

Run 1 mile

[Continued on next page]

Pull-Up x1; Push-Ups x2; Sit-Ups x 3; Pyramid from 10–6 (perform dynamic stretches for 25 meters after each set)

Run 1 mile

Pull-Up x1; Push-Ups x2; Sit-Ups x 3; Pyramid from 5–1 (perform dynamic stretches for 25 meters after each set)

Optional: If 1-10-1 is too easy, keep going up the pyramid to stop at 15 or 20 sets and double your volume of PT exercises.

#10
PST PRACTICE

Warm-up 5–10 minutes: your choice

Push-Ups – 2 minutes
Sit-Ups – 2 minutes
Pull-Ups – max

Run 1.5 miles timed

Rest 5 minutes

Run 1.5 mile timed

Push-Ups – 2 minutes
Sit-Ups – 2 minutes
Pull-Ups – max

[Continued on next page]

500 yard swim timed

Push-Ups – 2 minutes

Sit-Ups – 2 minutes

Pull-Ups – max effort (on pool deck if
   possible)

500 yard swim timed

If you don't have a pool, replace
   swimming with running or
   rucking for another 20–30
   minutes

#11
RUN AND PT PYRAMID PLUS

Warm-up: Run 1 mile

Warm-up: Pull-Up/Run/Push-Ups Pyramid 1–10

1 Pull-Up; Run 30 meters; 1 Push-Up; 2 Pull-Ups; Run 30 meters; 2 Push-Ups…up to 10/10 with runs/dynamic stretches in between

Repeat 5 times

Pull-Ups – max

Non-stop Push-Ups – max; stop when you have to rest

Sit-Ups – 1 minute

Push Press – max reps OR Hand Stand Push-Ups

[Continued on next page]

Run 400 meter sprint/400 meter jog (any order)

Swim 500 meter warm-up

Repeat 10 times

50 meter sprint – FREE

50 meter CSS – easy pace

Rest 1 minute treading water no hands

#12
RUN AND UPPER BODY
PT TEST TRAINING

1 mile jog warm-up/stretch

1 mile for time

Max Pull-Ups

Max Push-Ups – 1 minute

Max Sit-Ups – 1 minute

Repeat 3 times

   1 mile run, fast pace; shoot for 1
      mile run time above

   - Pull-Ups

   - Push-Ups

   - Sit-Ups

   - Plank Pose – 1 minute

[Continued on next page]

Repeat 5 times

Swim 250 yards using freestyle or CSS

Rest with 50 Flutterkicks and 50 Leg Levers

#13
RUN PT SUPER SETS WITH COOL-DOWN SWIM

Warm up with 1 mile short run

Repeat 10 times
Jumping Jacks (10)
Push-Ups (10)

Repeat 5–10 times
Run ¼ mile
Pull-Ups 5–10
Push-Ups 10–20
Sit-Ups 10–20
Dips – 10+
Plank Pose – 1 minute

[Continued on next page]

*Add in some TRX Push-Ups, TRX Rollouts (for planks), or TRX Rows for Pull-Ups options if needed.

Swim 500 meters timed, any stroke

Tread water (no hands) – 5 minutes

Swim 500 meters timed

#14
PT SUPER SET WITH RUN
AND SWIM PT

1 mile warm-up run or 10 minute bike/stretch

Repeat 4 times

½ mile at goal 1.5–2 mile timed run

Rest with Flutterkicks (50)

PT Super Set

Repeat 5 times

Pull-Ups 5–10 reps (sub max effort, do not fail)

Push-Ups – 20

Sit-Ups – 25 in 30 seconds

[Continued on next page]

Swim option:

Repeat 5 times

150 meters timed CSS

150 meters hypox freestyle at 8–10 strokes per breath

#15
20-MINUTE CARDIO SETS PLUS PT

Pick one of the following cardio options to do for 80 minutes, or do a mix of any/all for 20 minutes each. Every 20 minutes, stop and do the corresponding circuit for that cardio option.

Run 20 minutes timed

Max Pull-Ups, Max Push-Ups, Max Sit-Ups

Bike pyramid – 20 minutes

Max Pull-Ups, Max Push-Ups 2 minutes, Plank Pose – 2 minutes

Ruck 30-40# – 20 minutes

[Continued on next page]

Max Pull-Ups, Push-Ups, Plank Pose with backpack – 2 minutes

Swim – 20 minutes

How far do you get with fins? Without fins?

#16
NAVY SEAL PFT PLUS

When you're training for a specific test, it is always a good idea to make the test into a workout. If you are not assessing your progress, you are shooting in the dark. Plus, it is always a great workout regardless of your goals.

500 yard swim

Rest 10 minutes

Push-Ups – 2 minutes

Rest 2 minutes

Sit-Ups – 2 minutes

Rest 2 minutes

Pull-Ups – max effort

[Continued on next page]

PFT Transition:

Rest 10 minutes. Use the first 5 minutes to get the blood back to your legs by doing a short run of ¼ mile, shaking out your arms while you run and loosening your chest and shoulders. Spend the last five minutes stretching your legs with dynamic and static stretches prior to your run.

1.5 mile timed run

Go back to pool

5 x 100 meter swims at goal pace (i.e., 50 second 50 meters for 500 meters)

Rest 30 seconds

10 x 50 meters at goal pace for 500 meters

Rest with 30 seconds; tread with no hands

#17
8-COUNT PUSH-UP (OR BURPEE)/PULL-UPS PYRAMID

Run 2 miles

Do 1 Pull-Up; run 25 meters to an area to do Burpees or 8-count Push-Ups; do one 8-count Push-Up

Run 25 meters back to Pull-Up bar and do 2 Pull-Ups; run 25 meters; do two 8-count Push-Ups. Keep doing this, climbing each set until you fail at Pull-Ups, then repeat in reverse order.

Run 2 miles

*This is best if you have an outdoor pull-up bar or a pull-up bar in an open area like a basketball court. I usually do this one at a park or playground with monkey bars and a place to run a short distance.

#18
100-200-300 WORKOUT

Pick three calisthenics and do them for the prescribed repetitions. You can break them up into multiple sub-max effort sets, pyramids, or try to hit the numbers in as few sets as possible. One of these classic workouts is perfect for PT testing:

1.5 mile warm-up run

100 Pull-Ups
200 Push-Ups
300 Sit-Ups

1.5 mile cool-down run

*Option: Replace the 300 Sit-Ups with 300 squats for a Murph Workout.

#19
RUN AND PT MIX
(PUSH/PULL/PACED RUN)

Repeat 5 times

Pull-Ups – max effort

Push-Ups – max effort for 1 minute

400 meters at goal mile pace

400 meters at easy pace for recovery

#20
BURPEE PYRAMID WARM-UP WITH RUN/PT MIX

Warm up 5–10 minutes with Burpee pyramid 1–10 with 25 meters dynamic stretches in between

2 mile run, fast

Repeat 4 times

Run 400 meters at faster-than-goal pace

Push-Ups (20)

Sit-Ups (20)

2 mile run, fast

[Continued on next page]

Repeat 4 times

Run 400 meters at goal mile pace

Push-Ups (20)

Sit-Ups (20)

100 Pull-Ups any way you can, spread throughout the day if needed

#21
RUN AND PULL-UPS DAY

Pull-Ups 2-4-6-8-10

Stretch legs to prep for run in between.

Repeat 5 times

Run 1 mile

Max Pull-Ups

Swim Workout:

500 meters timed

5 x 100 meters skip breathing (also known as hypoxic swimming) at 8–10 strokes per breath

5 x 25 meters underwater

Rest 20 seconds

*You should never swim alone or without a lifeguard, especially when skip breathing or practicing underwater swims.

#22
RUN AND PULL-UPS/PUSH-UPS

Pull-Ups 2-4-6-8-10

Stretch legs to prep for run in between.

Repeat 3–4 times

Run 1 mile

Max Pull-Ups

Max Push-Ups and 1 minute Sit-Ups or TRX Atomic Push-Ups. Try to double your Pull-Up reps each set

Ruck or swim with fins, total time 30–45 minutes (your choice).

#23
BURPEE/PULL-UP PYRAMID

1.5 mile warm-up run

1–20 Pyramid (just up the pyramid)
= 210 Pull-Ups/Burpees with 25
meter runs in between Pull-Up
bar and Burpee area

1-10-1 Pyramid = 100 Pull-Ups/
Burpees (your choice depending
upon your time and abilities)

Run 1.5 mile cool-down

#24
WEAKNESS FOCUS
(RUN OR PT CHOICES)

Run 1 mile warm-up

Warm up with 1-5 Pull-Up/Push-Up
pyramid with 25 meters run in
between

PT Weakness x5

Pull-Ups – max effort

Push-Ups – max 1 minute

Push Press – max (40–50 pounds)

Dips – max effort

Run ¼ mile at goal mile pace

OR

Run Weakness x 5

Run 1 mile at goal pace for timed runs

Push-Ups – 20

Pull-Ups –10–20

Push Press – 20 (40–50 pounds)

Dip –10–20

Cool down with 5-1 Pull-Up/Push-Up Pyramid with 25 meter runs in between

Run 1 mile cool-down

#25
RUN HILLS AND INTERVALS MIXED WITH PT

Run 2 miles

Run hills or ¼ mile laps mixed with
  bleachers or stairs for 5 minutes

Repeat as many times as you can for
  30 minutes, but mix 25 Push-Ups
  each set

Run 2 miles but accumulate 100
  Burpees (break up as desired)

100 Pull-Ups any way you can, spread
  throughout the day if needed

Tread water (no hands) 15 minutes,
  all kicks practiced (scissor,
  flutterkick, breast, egg beater)

#26
100 REPS WORKOUT

1 mile easy run

100 Pull-Ups
100 Push-Ups
100 Sit-Ups

1 mile run

100 Dips
100 Flutterkicks
100 Push Press

1 mile run with sandbag or ruck

1 mile easy run without weight

#27
5 MINUTES ON/5 MINUTES OFF

Repeat 5 minute run and 5 minute PT sets until you get 100, 200, 300

Run 5 minutes, then PT or lift 5 minutes. Repeat until done with reps, but *only* take 5 minute sets to accomplish reps of Pull-Ups, Push-Ups, abs of choice

Total numbers:

100 Pull-Ups

200 Push-Ups OR 100 Bench Press (135 pounds) and 100 Push-Ups

300 abs: 100 Flutterkicks, 100 Leg Levers, 100 Scissors

Complete in circuit fashion with max rep sets until reps are reached, but only in 5 minute sets

#28
TEN PT SUPER SETS

Repeat 10 times

Pull-Ups – 10

Push-Ups – 25

Abs of choice (50) OR Plank Pose –
　　1 minute

Dips – 20

3 mile run, timed

#29
RUN AND SWIM PT

5 minutes warm-up/stretch

100 Pull-Ups any way you can, rest as
   needed

Mix abs of choice and Lightweight
   Shoulder Workout in between
   sets

Run 3 mile test

Swim

Repeat 10–20 times

100 meters CSS

20 Push-Ups

20 abs of choice (add in 1 minute
   Plank Pose on odd sets)

#30
SWIM PT

Repeat 10 times

100 meter free hypox at 8–10 strokes per breath

50 meter CSS at goal pace

Push-Ups – 20

Sit-Ups – 20

Flutterkicks – 20

Plank Pose – 1 minute

#31
SWIM/PLANK WORKOUT

Repeat 5 times

Swim 200 meters

Tread for as long as it takes to swim 200 meters

Push-Ups and Plank Pose for the time it takes to swim 200 meters

#32
RUN OR SWIM PT

15 minutes run, bike, or elliptical warm-up/stretch

Swim or Run PT

500 meter swim or

1 mile run

Repeat 5 times

Run or swim 200 meters

Push-Ups – 1 minute

Plank Pose – 1 minute

Abs of choice – 1 minute

15 minutes run, bike, swim, or elliptical cool-down/stretch

#33
SPARTAN RUN/PT

5 minutes warm-up/stretch

Spartan run

Run 15 minutes

100 Push-Ups

100 abs of choice

Run 15 minutes

75 Push-Ups

200 abs of choice

Run 15 minutes

50 Push-Ups

300 abs of choice

Run 20 minutes

[Continued on next page]

If using Plank Pose for your abs of choice, 1 second = 1 rep

Mix some 8-count Body Builders, Dive Bombers, and Burpees into the Push-Up section and do the Push-Ups anyway you can.

#34
SUPERSET WORKOUT
WITH RUNS

Warm up with 1 mile short run or 10 minutes bike or elliptical

Repeat 10 times
Jumping Jacks – 10
Push-Ups – 10

PT Super Set:
Repeat 5–10 times
Run ¼ mile
Pull-Ups – 5–10
Push-Ups – 10–20
Sit-Ups – 10–20
Dips – 10+

[Continued on next page]

Plank Pose – 1 minute

*Add in some TRX Push-Ups, TRX Rollouts, or TRX Rows for ab options if needed

Run 1 mile cool-down or bike/elliptical for 10 minutes, easy pace

#35
RUN AND PT MIX
(PUSH/PULL/SPRINT)

Repeat 5 times

Pull-Ups – max effort

Push-Ups – max effort for 1 minute

50 meter easy jog

100 meter sprint

50 meter easy jog

100 meter sprint

#36
THE UBRR
(UPPER BODY ROUND ROBIN)

Warm up with 5 minutes jogging, dynamic stretches, and static stretches

1 minute Push-Ups (minimum 40)

1 minute Sit-Ups (minimum 40)

Pull-Ups (minimum 6), not timed

Dips (minimum 6), not timed

Bench Press – 80 percent of body weight (minimum 6), not timed

20 foot rope climb in body armor or weight vest (just once, pass or fail event)

1 minute Kip-Ups (minimum 6), hang from pull-up bar and bring feet to bar

- 4 x 25 meter shuttle run (max 24 seconds)
- 5 mile run (max 40 minutes) or 5 mile ruck march (75 minutes max, 45 pounds dry weight)
- Additional 500 meters swim test (optional)

#37
RUN AND UPPER BODY PT CHALLENGE

Warm-up/stretch

Pull-Ups: 2-4-6-8-10 (stretch legs in between sets)

2 mile run

Repeat 6 times

Pull-Ups – max

TRX Atomic Push-Ups – max effort OR Regular Push-Ups (no TRX)

Sit-Ups – 1 minute

Run ¼ mile at goal mile pace

#38
BRUTAL RUN AND BURPEE PT

Run 1.5 minutes; Burpees 1.5
  minutes; max Pull-Ups; max Dips

Run 3 minutes; Burpees 3 minutes;
  max Pull-Ups; max Dips

Run 4.5 minutes; Burpees 4.5
  minutes; max Pull-Ups; max Dips

Shoot for ¼ mile for every 90 second
  run pace

#39
RUN AND PT CHALLENGE

Warm up with 5 minutes of jogging

Pull-Ups: 2-4-6-8-10 (do 10 Push-Ups and 10 Sit-Ups in between Pull-Ups)

Repeat 3 times

Push-Ups – 1 minute

Sit-Ups – 1 minute

Pull-Ups – max

Dips – max

1 mile run

Repeat 2 times

TRX Push-Ups or elevated Push-Ups – max

Sit-Ups – 1 minute

Weighted Pull-Ups – max effort (10–20 pounds)

Dips – max

4 x 25 meters shuttle run

Swim Cool-Down Option

Swim 500 meters

Plank Pose – 1 minute

Flutterkicks 1 minute

Swim 500 meters with fins

#40
BIG RUN AND PT WORKOUT SETS

Warm up with 5 minutes of jogging

Pull-Ups: 2-4-6-8-10 (do 10 Push-Ups and 10 Sit-Ups in between Pull-Ups)

Repeat 3 times

Run 2 miles

Pull-Ups – max

Dips – max

Repeat 5 times

Swim 200 meters

Push-Ups – 1 minute

Sit-Ups – 1 minute

Plank Pose – 1 minute

Swim or Run PT

Repeat 6 times

100 meters sprint swim or 200 meters sprint running

25 Push-Ups

25 abs of choice or 30 seconds Plank Pose

#41
RUN/PT AND SWIM PT

Repeat 4–5 times

Pull-Ups – max effort

Push-Ups – 50

Sit-Ups – 50

Dips – 25

Run 1 mile fast

Ruck or Swim 30 minutes: Shoot for 2–3 mile ruck or at least 1500 meters swim, with or without fins

#42
100 METERS BURPEE PYRAMID PLUS PT PYRAMID

Do 1 Burpee, get up and run 100 yards; do 2 Burpees, run 100 yards; do 3 Burpees, run 100 yards, etc. Keep going until you run out of time or energy. Goal: Get up to 25 sets in 45–50 minutes.

1 mile timed run after completed

PT Pyramid: Pull-Up x1, Dip x2, Sit-Up or abs of choice x 5 (no Push-Ups)

How high can you go up the pyramid until you fail at both Pull-Ups and Dips?

1 mile cool-down run

#43
RUN AND UPPER BODY PT

Run 1.5 mile warm-up jog

Repeat 5 times

Max Pull-Ups, run 200 yards

Max Push-Ups (1 minute), run 200 yards

Sit-Ups or Flutterkicks – 2 minutes

*Goal: Can you get 100 Pull-Ups in 5 sets?

Run 1.5 mile cool-down jog

Lower Body
Calisthenics and Cardio

#44
TRACK RUN AND LEG PT

1 mile warm-up jog or 5 minutes bike/stretch

1 mile timed run

Repeat 10 times

¼ mile at goal mile pace (for example: 6-minute mile = ¼ mile in 90 seconds)

Rest with 20 leg/ab exercises of your choice: Squats, Lunges, Heel Raises, Flutterkicks, Leg Levers, Sit-Ups, etc.

Option for ¼s:

If you want some jog/sprint combos, try jogging the corners of the track and sprinting the straights (100 meters sprint; 100 meters jog; 100 meters sprint; 100 meters jog)

Swim (in pool) for cool-down

5 x 100 meter swims at goal pace (swim each 100 meters at your goal 500 meters pace; for example: 50 meters in 50 seconds = 8:20 500 meters pace)

Rest 30 seconds

10 x 50 meters at goal pace for 500 meters (swim with fins if you prefer)

#45
LEG PT AND CARDIO/ NON-IMPACT OPTION

Repeat 5 times

Bike/elliptical 5 minutes fast (Tabata interval)

Air Squats – 20

Air Lunges – 10/leg

Dead Lift – 5 (with barbells, dumbbells, or sandbag)

Front Squats – 5 (with barbells, dumbbells, or sandbag)

Run ½ mile in place of Tabata interval (if you prefer to run) and do leg PT/lift

Ruck 2 miles or swim (with fins) 1000 meters to top off leg day

Do dynamic stretches in pool (chest deep water) – 5 minutes (Butt Kickers, Leg Swings, Frankenstein Kicks, etc.)

#46
FAST RUNS AND LEG PT

Run 15–20 minutes
How far do you get?

Repeat 6 times
Run 200 meters fast
Squats – 20

Repeat 6 times
Run 400 meters fast
Lunges – 10/leg

#47
RUCK AND LEG DAY

Ruck 60 minutes, stopping every 10 minutes to do 20 squats and 10 lunges per leg

Swim 1500 meters (with fins) or 20 minutes bike pyramid if no pool is available

#48
LEG DAY AND CARDIO INTERVALS

Squat/Run Pyramid 1–20: Run 25 meters, do 1 Squat; run 25 meters, do 2 Squats…up to 20 Squats. You can also do dynamic stretches in between Squat sets (Butt Kickers, Leg Swings, other stretches)

Squat/Stair Pyramid 1–10: Do the same pyramid as above but run up/down a flight of steps in between 1–10 sets; 1 squat, up/down flight of steps; 2 squats, up/down flight of steps…until you complete 10 sets.

Repeat 4 times

Easy cardio – 5 minutes

Squats – 5–10 (with weight: barbell, kettlebell, or dumbbells)

Dead Lift – 5 (with weight: barbell, kettlebell, or dumbbells)

Lunges – 10/leg (no weight)

Farmer Walk – 3 (holding 25–40 pound dumbbell in one hand, going up/down flight of steps)

Swim 20–30 minutes with fins OR bike pyramid*

*Bike pyramid: Make each minute harder by adding a level of resistance (or two) each minute for 10–15 minutes, then repeat in reverse order. Keep RPMs at 70–90.

#49
TRACK AND PT WORKOUT
(SPEED AND PACE DRILLS)

¼ mile warm-up

Squats – 20

Half Squats – 20 (all the way down, halfway up)

Lunges – 10/leg

Butt Kickers – 30 seconds

Leg Swings – 10/leg

Light stretch

Repeat 4 times

¼ mile run at goal pace for 1.5 mile timed runs

Rest with 25 abs of choice

Repeat 4 times

¼ mile of jogging on curves, sprinting on straights on track or 100 meters jog/100 meters sprint x 2

Rest with Butt Kickers or Leg Swings

Repeat 16 times

100 meters sprint: build up to full speed at the 50 meter mark

Rest with 20 Push-Ups/20 Squats or Lunges

Swim or Bike 30 minutes

Every 5 minutes, stop and do max Push-Ups and Flutterkicks (1 minute each). Do Pull-Ups (max reps) if a pull-up bar is available.

#50
SPEC OPS LEG DAY

Ruck 2 miles at moderate pace with 50 pound backpack (or 25 percent of your bodyweight)

Run 2 miles but in interval/leg PT mix:

Jog – 50 meters

Sprint – 100 meters

Squats – 20

Swim and Leg PT

Swim 500 meter warm-up without fins

Mix in 20 lunges on pool deck every 100 meters (10/leg)

Swim with fins – 1000 meters

Tread water (no hands) 15 minutes: all kicks practiced (scissor, flutterkick, breast, and egg beater)

#51
RUN AND LEG PT

Run 1 mile warm-up/stretch

Run hills, steps, bleachers, sand, etc. for 30 minutes, stopping every 5 minutes to do 20 squats and 10 lunges.

Run 1 mile cool-down

#52
LOWER BODY PT

Repeat 4 times
With backpack:
Ruck with 50 pounds – 10 minutes
Squats – 25
Lunges – 10–15/leg
Heel Raises – 20

Core PT Section

Repeat 3 times
Flutterkicks – 50
Leg Levers – 50
Atomic Sit-Ups – 25

Run 3 miles

#53
TRACK LEG AND CORE WORKOUT

¼ mile warm-up/stretch

Repeat 12 times

¼ mile at goal mile pace (for example: 6-minute mile = ¼ mile in 90 seconds)

Pick 1 leg exercise plus 1 ab exercise in between each ¼ mile: 1 minute each

Bring Weights to Track

Kettlebell Cleans – 1 minute

Kettlebell Goblet Squats – 1 minute

Dumbbell Thrusters – 1 minute

Squats – 1 minute

Lunges – 1 minute (30 seconds/leg)

1 minute of core: Sit-Ups, Crunches, Plank Pose, Flutterkicks, Leg Levers

Swim Cool-Down

1000 meters with fins

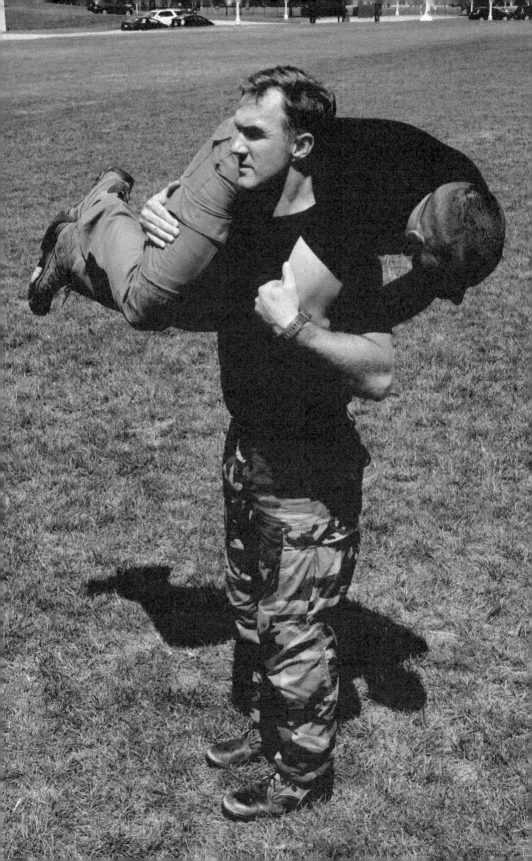

Full Body Calisthenics/ Resistance and Cardio

#54
RUN WARM-UP WITH PT PYRAMID MAX EFFORT/RUN COOL-DOWN

Run 1.5 mile

Push-Up/Pull-Ups Pyramid 1-15 or 20

1 Push-Up, run 50 meters; 1 Pull-Up, run 50 meters; 2 Pull-Ups, run 50 meters; 2 Pull-Ups, run 50 meters…keep going until 15–20 sets

If you can get above 10, do not repeat in reverse order. Keep going up the pyramid until you fail at any exercise. If you fail at 10 or less sets, repeat in reverse order.

Run 50 meters: this workout is best done outside where you have a pull-up bar in a field or open space.

For extra credit, try adding other forms of travel to make the workout tougher or easier:

Tougher ideas: Fireman Carry, Bear Crawls, Crab Walks, Farmer Walks, Walking Lunges, etc.

Easier ideas: Various dynamic stretches (Butt Kickers, Frankenstein Walks, High Knees, etc.)

Run 1.5 mile

#55
RUN AND LEG PT WITH LIFTS

¼ mile warm-up

Squats – 20

Half Squats – 20

Lunges – 10/leg

Stretch as needed

Bring 45 pound dumbbell or plate to
track.

Repeat 12 times

¼ mile run at goal pace for 1.5–2 mile
timed runs

Rest with 20 reps of Wood Chopper
Squats or Lunges, 100 yard
Farmer Walks, or 10 Turkish Get-
Ups

Run or Bike 30 minutes

Every 5 minutes, stop and do max Pull-Ups and Flutterkicks – 1 minute each

How many Pull-Ups can you get in 5 sets (above)?

#56
RUN AND SWIM SKILLS

½ mile warm-up/stretch

Run/Burpee Ladder

Run 100 yards, 1 Burpee; run 100 yards, 2 Burpees; run 100 yards, 3 Burpees…keep going up to 20

½ mile cool-down

Swim Skills

Repeat 10 times

Swim 100 meters

Tread water with no hands, bob, and float (drown-proofing test events) for the time it takes to swim 100 meters

Run #2

3 mile run

#57
DEVIL'S MILE PREP

Run ½ mile

200 yards Bear Crawl

¼ mile run

200 yards Lunges

¼ mile run

200 yards Burpee Forward Jump

¼ mile run

200 yard Farmer Walk or Fireman
  Carry (100 yards each)

¼ mile run

Run ½ mile easy

50 Pull-Ups in as few sets as possible

#58
TRACK/FIELD WORKOUT

Repeat 4 times

Run ¼ mile at goal timed run pace (for example: 6-minute mile = ¼ mile in 90 seconds)

100 yards of Burpee/Broad Jumps*

***Burpee Broad Jump: drop forward to Push-Up position, stand back up, jump forward, repeat for 100 yards**

Pull-Ups/Dips/Abs

Pull-Ups – 100

Dips – 150

Abs – 200 anyway you can

[Continued on next page]

Swim or Bike Workout
20–30 minutes
How far do you get?

#59
RUN INTERVALS AND WEIGHTS PT

Run/warm-up 10 minutes

Run ¼ mile at goal pace OR bike 2 minutes

Burpees – 90 seconds

Run ¼ mile

Thrusters (with dumbbells 20–40 pounds) – 90 seconds

Run ¼ mile

Box Jumps – 90 seconds

Run ¼ mile

Kettlebell Swings (30–40 pounds) – 90 seconds

Run ¼ mile

[Continued on next page]

Swim, Run, or Bike PT

Swim, run, or bike 2 minutes

Push-Ups – 50

Abs – 50

Swim, run, or bike 4 minutes

Max Push-Ups/Abs – 50 OR Plank
Pose – 1 minute

Swim, run, or bike 6 minutes

Max Push-Ups/Abs – 50 OR Plank
Pose – 1 minute

Swim, run, or bike 8 minutes

20 Push-Ups/10 Pull-Ups/10 Dips/
Plank Pose – 1 minute

Cool-down: swim, run, or bike 10
minutes/stretch

#60
RUN AND PT WORKOUT

Warm up 5 minutes jog/stretch

Pull-Ups 2-4-6-8-10: Do 10 Push-Ups/10 Sit-Ups in between Pull-Ups

Repeat 5 times

1 mile run

Pull-Ups – max

Push-Ups – max effort OR use TRX and try to double your Pull-Up score with Atomic Push-Ups

Sit-Ups – 1 minute

Flutterkicks – 1 minute

Kettlebell Swings – 1 minute

#61
RUN AND FULL BODY PT (WITH DBS, KETTLEBELLS, OR SANDBAGS)

Warm up 5 minutes jog/stretch

Pull-Ups 2-4-6-8-10

Do 10 Push-Ups/10 Sit-Ups in between Pull-Ups

Repeat 4 times

1 mile run

Pull-Ups – max

Box Jumps – 1 minute

Kettlebell Swings – 1 minute

Burpees – 1 minute

Thrusters (with dumbbells or barbells, total weight 75–100 pounds) – 1 minute

#62
SANDBABY 500 WITH KETTLEBELL AND TRX

Pull-Ups – 100

Push Press – 100 (with weights*)

TRX Atomic Push-Ups – 100

Squats – 100 (with weights*)

Kettlebell Swings – 100

*Use 40–50 pound weights for Squats and Push Press (sandbag, kettlebell, etc.)

Run through the workout in circuit fashion, but every time you total 100 reps, stop and run a mile.

With a total of 500 reps in this workout you will run 4 miles total.

[Continued on next page]

Ruck or swim 30 minutes: Shoot for 2–3 mile ruck or at least 1500 meters swim, with or without fins.

#63
DEVILS MILE

Progress with this one over time.

Do a few workouts where you build up from 100 meter and 200 meter exercises before tackling the full Devil's Mile:

1 mile warm-up jog

400 meters Bear Crawl

400 meters Walking Lunges

400 meters Fireman Carry*

400 meters Burpee Jump or Forward Roll

[Continued on next page]

*Replacement options:
- Sandbag Carry for Fireman Carry
- Farmer Walk for Fireman Carry

Run 2 miles cool-down

#64
RUN AND FULL BODY PT COMBO

Run 1.5 mile warm-up jog

Repeat 5 times

Run 200 meters fast

Pull-Ups – Max

Fireman Carry – 100 meters OR Body Drags – 50 meters

Push-Ups – 1 minute

Flutterkicks – 1 minute

The goal is to get 100 Pull-Ups in 5 sets or less; keep going until you get 100 Pull-Ups.

Run 1.5 mile cool-down jog

#65
RUN AND FULL BODY
AND SWIM PT

Run ¼ mile warm-up/stretch

**Walking Lunges – 30 steps OR 30
Frog Hops (broad jumps)**

Run ½ mile

Stretch

**Walking Lunges – 30 steps OR 30
Frog Hops**

Run ¾ mile

Stretch

**Walking Lunges – 30 steps OR 30
Frog Hops**

Run ½ mile timed

Stretch

Run ¼ mile at goal 1.5 mile timed run
   pace

Pull-Ups

Max reps x 5 sets

Rest with Push-Ups x 2 # of Pull-Up
   you've done

(Add TRX Atomic Push-Ups if you
   have a TRX)

Swim Workout

Repeat 3 times

500 yards at 8–9 strokes per breath
   freestyle

Push-Ups – 1 minute

Sit-Ups – 1 minute

Tread water 1 minute (no hands)

#66
INTERVAL RUN AND SWIM WITH UPPER BODY AND LEG PT

Easy jog warm-up 5 minutes

Repeat 4 times
Run ¼ mile fast
Walk 100 meters for rest

1 minute of each
Pull-Ups – max
Box Jumps – max OR Frog Hops
8 count Push-Ups or Burpees
Wood Chopper Squats OR Kettlebell Swings
Swim 500 meters warm-up plus 1000 meters with fins for time

#67
BURPEE/LEG AND CORE PT

Repeat 5 times

Run 50 meters

Burpees – 10

Flutterkicks – 25

Repeat 5 times

Fireman Carry – 50 meters

Burpees – 10

Leg Levers – 25

Repeat 5 times

Bear Crawl – 50 meters

Burpees – 10

Scissors – 25

[Continued on next page]

Repeat 5 times

Burpee/Broad Jump for 50 meters

50 abs of choice

#68
8 COUNT BODY BUILDER (OR BURPEE)/PULL-UP PYRAMID

1 mile warm-up run or 10 minute bike

1 Pull-Up, run 25 meters; 1 Burpee, run 25 meters; 2 Pull-Ups, run 25 meters; 2 Burpees, run 25 meters…keep going up until you fail at Pull-Ups

If under 10 sets, then repeat in reverse order. If over 10 sets, just keep going up. How high can you get?

Get creative on even sets: Bear Crawl, Low Crawl, Fireman Carry with partner or sandbag, Body Drags, Lunges, or other moving exercise of your choice. Try not to repeat the same one too many times.

Run 2 miles timed

#69
RUN AND FULL BODY PT

1 mile run OR 10 minute warm-up on bike or elliptical or other

Repeat 6 times

Run ¼ mile 10 seconds faster than 1.5 mile pace

Wood Chopper Squats or Kettlebell Swings – 20

Wood Chopper Lunges – 10/leg

Box Jumps – 10–15 OR Stair climbs/ bleacher run for 1 minute

Ruck 2 miles for time with 30–40 pounds

Swim with fins for 1000 meters or bike pyramid for 20 minutes

#70
100, 200, 300+ RUN AND LEG PT

Do in as few sets as possible:

100 Pull-Ups*

200 Push-Ups

300 Sit-Ups

Alternate max reps sets of each exercise, keeping track of total reps each cycle. Stop when you reach all the goal numbers with no rest other than sips of water and stretching.

*Use Pulldowns or Knee Push-Ups when you fail at Pull-Ups/Push-Ups. You can also add in Crunches/Plank if you fail at Sit-Ups.

[Continued on next page]

Repeat 6 times

¼ mile at goal 1.5 mile pace

In between ¼ mile runs do one of the following each time:

100 yard Bear Crawl

100 yard Lunges

100 yard Burpee Jumps

50 yard Fireman Carry

100 yard Farmer Walk With 45 pounds in one hand

100 yard Crab Walk

#71
COMBO 100, 200, 300
WORKOUT

1 mile easy run

100 Pull-Ups*
200 Push-Ups

1 mile run with sandbag or ruck

100 Push Press
200 Lunges (100/leg chest carry
      weight)
150 Sit-Ups/Chest Carry
150 Squat Shoulder Carry

1 mile run with sandbag or ruck

[Continued on next page]

1 mile easy run without weight

*If you cannot do 100 Pull-Ups in 5–6
    sets, add in Pulldowns or Rows
    to get to 100 reps faster

#72
WARM-UP SQUAT/PUSH-UP/ RUN PYRAMID 1-10

Run 25 meters, 1 Squat, 1 Push-Up; run 25 meters, 2 Squats, 2 Push-Ups…keep going up to 10 and then stop.

Repeat 5 times

Pull-Ups – max

TRX Push-Ups OR regular Push-Ups – max

TRX Rollouts – 10–15 OR Plank Pose – 1 minute

Bear Crawls – 25 meters

[Continued on next page]

Repeat 5 times

Squats – max 1 minute (shoulder carry sandbag or backpack)

Dips – max

Sit-Ups – 1 minute

Bear Crawls – 25 meters

Run 3 miles or swim 500 meters for warm-up

Repeat 10 times

200 meters fast, any stroke

Rest with tread, bounce, float – 1 minute each set

#73
BURPEE PYRAMID WITH SPARTAN RUN/PT

Warm up 5 minutes jog

Burpee Pyramid

1 Burpee, run 100 meters; 2 Burpees, run 100 meters; 3 Burpees, run 100 meters...on your fifth set, do max Pull-Ups and then:

6 Burpees, run 100 meters...keep going to 10, then do max Pull-Ups

Spartan Run/PT

¼ mile run at goal mile pace

Push Press – 50

¼ mile run at goal mile pace

[Continued on next page]

Kettlebell Swings – 50

¼ mile run at goal mile pace

Pull-Ups – 50

¼ mile run at goal mile pace

Walking Lunges – 50 steps

¼ mile run at goal mile pace

Plank Pose – 2 Minutes

¼ mile at goal mile pace

Swim 30 minutes

How far do you get? Shoot for 30+ laps minimum, any stroke OR ruck 30 minutes for distance

#74
BURPEE PYRAMID WITH RUN AND STAIR CRAWLS

Burpee Pyramid 1–5

1 Burpee, run 30 meters; 2 Burpees, run 30 meters; 3 Burpees, run 30 meters; 4 Burpees, run 30 meters; 5 Burpees, run 30 meters

Dips – max effort

Pull-Ups – max effort

Stair Crawls down/up OR Bear Crawl – 50 meters

[Continued on next page]

Burpee Pyramid 6–10

Dips – max effort

Pull-Ups – max effort

Stair Crawls down/up OR Bear Crawl – 50 meters

Burpee Pyramid 10–6 (or advanced 11–15)

Dips – max effort

Pull-Ups – max effort

Stair Crawls down/up OR Bear Crawl – 50 meters

Burpee Pyramid 5–1 (or advanced 16–20)

Dips – max effort

Pull-Ups – max effort

Stair Crawls down/up OR Bear Crawl – 50 meters

#75
100, 200, 300, 400, 500
WORKOUT

Warm up with Burpee Pyramid run:
1 Burpee, run 50 meters; 2
Burpees, run 50 meters…stop
at 10

Stair Crawls up/down OR Bear Crawl
– 50 meters

Total reps, done any way you want:

100 pull (Pull-Ups, Pulldowns,
Rows, etc.)

200 push: (Burpees count as 100, so
add 100 reps of Bench Press,
Dips, Military Push-Ups, or any
combo of 100)

300 Squats (no weights)

[Continued on next page]

400 abs of choice

500 seconds Plank Pose

Stair Crawls down/up OR Bear Crawl – 50 meters

Cool down Burpees

9 Burpees, run 50 meters; 8 Burpees, run 50 meters…repeat and return to 1 for 100 total Burpees

Swim

500 meters timed CSS

400 meters hypox at 8–10 strokes per breath

300 meters = 3 x 100 meters goal pace CSS

200 meters CSS sprint

100 meters sprint any stroke

500 meters cool-down with fins

#76
BLUE FALCON WORKOUT

This workout is best if you have a buddy to do exercises with you.

Run 1 mile warm-up

100 meters Bear Crawl/100 Push Press (40 pounds)

100 meters Overhead Walking Lunges (40 pounds)/100 Sit-Ups (40 pounds)

100 meters Burpee Jump/100 Flutterkicks

100 meters Farmer Walk (40 pounds dumbbell/100 squats)

100 meters Fireman Carry or 400 meters sandbag run/100 Kettlebell Swings

[Continued on next page]

100 meters sandbag head carry (place sandbag on your head)/100 Burpees

Without buddy: Go through all exercises like a circuit. Do not move onto the next exercise until 100 reps or 100 meters have been accomplished. Rest as needed.

With buddy: One person does the distance exercise and the other does the 100 rep exercise. The distance exerciser cannot finish that event until 100 reps have been completed by his buddy. Then switch exercises. The distance is capped at 200 meters; if distance gets to 200 meters, then the 100 reps can be stopped.

Run 1 mile with sandbag (40 pounds)

#77
100, 200, 300 LOG PT SIMULATION

1 mile run with sandbag (40 pounds)

100 Push Press

200 Walking Lunges (100/leg; Chest Carry 40 pound weight or sandbag)

300 = 150 squats + 150 Sit-Ups with 40 pound sandbag on shoulder or chest

1 mile run with sandbag (40 pounds)

#78
HELLACIOUS 100S

All exercises get 100 reps, rest as needed (make a circuit to keep moving)

Warm up with 1–10 Burpee pyramid with 25 meters dynamic stretch/run

100 Pull-Ups/Rows (if needed)

100 Push-Ups

100 Sit-Ups

100 Flutterkicks

100 Squats

100 Leg Levers

100 Lunges (50/leg)

100 Scissors

100 Dumbbell Bench Press (50 percent body weight)

100 Dumbbell or Sandbag Push Press (25–50 percent body weight)

End with 9–1 Burpee pyramid with 25 meters dynamic stretch/run = 100 Burpees

Run 2 miles

#79
HARD REVERSE PYRAMID

20-19-18-17-16: Push-Ups, Sit-Ups, Arm Haulers

Max Dips/Pull-Ups

15-14-13-12-11: Pull-Ups, Push-Ups, Sit-Ups

100 Flutterkicks (non-stop)

10-9-8-7-6: Pull-Ups, Bench Press, Push Press (50 percent up to BW)

Run 1 mile or bike 10 minutes

5-4-3-2-1 = 15 reps in one set: Pull-Ups, Push Press, MJDB #1 (OR Kettlebell Clean and Press)

#80
PUSH, PULL, CRAWLS

1–10 Burpee/Run 25 meters Pyramid

Bear Crawl – 50 meters

Dips – max

Repeat 3 times

Pull-Ups – max

Bench Press – 20 (50 percent body weight)

Bear Crawl – 50 Meters OR Dips – max

Repeat 3 times

Pull-Ups – max

Push Press – 20 (25–50 percent body weight)

Bear Crawl – 50 Meters OR Dips – max effort

Repeat 3 times

Pull-Ups – max

Push-Ups – max effort THEN Hold plank for 2 minutes

10–1 Burpee/Run 25 meters Pyramid

Run 1.5 miles timed

#81
RUN/CALISTHENICS AND KETTLEBELLS

Warm up with 5 minute jog/stretch

Repeat 4 times

Run 1 mile

Pull-Ups – max

Push-Ups – max

Plank Pose – 1 minute

Kettlebell Swings – 20

Push Press – 20 (with sandbag or kettlebell)

Box Jumps – 10

Flutterkicks – 50

Squats – 20

Lunges – 10/Leg

Ruck with 40 pounds or swim 30 minutes with fins for distance.

How far do you get?

#82
DEATH BY PUSH-UPS PLUS UPPER BODY PT/CARDIO

Warm up with 10 minutes run or bike to loosen shoulders, chest, and arms.

Death by Push-Ups 1–20: You are in the Push-Up or Plank Position for 20 minutes! You do one step of the pyramid every minute for 20 minutes. The first minute = 1 Push-Up, second minute = 2 Push-Ups, third minute = 3 Push-Ups…all the way up to 20 minutes = 20 Push-Ups. You can also do it in reverse order if you prefer. Try not to rest on your knees. Stay in Push-Up, Down Dog, or Up Dog yoga pose or Plank Pose the whole time.

Repeat 4 times

Pull-Ups – max effort (plus one
   negative)

Dumbbell Rows – 10/arm

Military Press – 10

Sit-Ups – 1 minute

Cardio – "rest" 3 minutes easy pace
   (run, bike, row, elliptical, etc.)

Optional swim or run workout

Swim 500 meters warm-up

Repeat 10 times

100 meters CSS or freestyle

Pull-Outs – 10 (pull body out of the
   pool as if you are doing a muscle
   up on the pool edge)

[Continued on next page]

If running:

Warm up with 1 mile jog

Repeat 6 times

¼ mile fast pace run

100 yard walk

#83
SEVEN SETS OF FIVE-MINUTE CIRCUITS

5 minutes bike or elliptical Tabata interval: 20 seconds fast/10 seconds easy

5 minutes Pull-Ups: rest as needed, max out (rest counts as total time)

5 minutes Push-Ups and Plank Pose: no resting on knees

5 minutes Kettlebell Swings/ Snatches/Clean Press: just keep it moving the whole time

[Continued on next page]

5 minutes Walking Lunges with 25 pounds Overhead Presses: rest weight on your head if you must (best weight is a sandbag)

5 minutes Flutterkicks: no placing feet on floor

5 minutes TRX: select as many exercises as you want, just keep moving with TRX for 5 minutes or pick something else if no TRX is available, like a jump rope, battle ropes, etc.

35 minutes run for max distance

35 minutes swim or ruck for max distance

#84
RUN AND LEG PT TRACK WORKOUT

Repeat 8 times

¼ mile at 90–100 seconds

Rest 45 seconds

Repeat 25 times

50 meters jog/50 meters sprint

Pick any exercise from below and do 25 reps in between each 50/50 meters:

Push-Ups (any type)

Sit-Ups

Crunches (any type)

Flutterkicks

[Continued on next page]

Leg Levers

Scissors

TRX (any exercise)

Squats, Lunges, or Heel Raises

Kettlebell Swings

Woodchoppers

8-count Push-Ups

Burpees

1 mile swim with fins or easy jog of
2–3 miles

#85
BUILD YOUR OWN PFT

Non-impact cardio

Pick one: 500 meters swim, 10 mile bike, 2000 meters row

Upper body

Pick two: Pull-Ups, Push-Ups, TRX Atomic Push-Ups, Bench Press (max reps bodyweight)

Abs

Pick two: Sit-Ups, Crunches, Flutterkicks, Plank Pose – 2 minutes

[Continued on next page]

Fast run

Pick one: 100 meters sprint, 300 meters sprint, 120 yard shuttle run (4 x 30), ¼ mile sprint, IL Agility Test

Longer run

Pick one: 1.5 mile timed run, 2 mile timed run, 3 mile timed run, 4 mile timed run

*Rest in between as long as you need

Cardio and Mobility: Run, Ruck, and/or Swim

#86
CARDIO ONLY DAY

Ruck or run 30–60 minutes

How far do you get?

Swim 30 minutes

How far do you get? If no pool is available, then bike or row for same time for max distance.

Swim or Ruck

500 meters swim with fins

Repeat 10 times (no fins)

100 meters free sprint, rest with easy 50 meters CSS

500 meters swim with fins

Or, if no pool is available, ruck 4 miles in under an hour with 40–50 pounds

#87
PACED RUNS AND SWIM TESTS

Jog 2 miles easy pace/stretch 5 minutes

Run up/down hills, stairs, or bleachers for 15 minutes

Run fast 2 miles

Swim Workout

500 meters without fins timed (free or CSS)

1000 meters with fins timed (free or CSS)

Tread water 10 minutes holding brick, weight, etc. (15–20 pounds) with fins

#88
RUN, SWIM, RUCK

3 miles run timed

500 meters swim timed (any stroke)

Repeat 10 times

50 meters freestyle at 8–10 strokes per breath (skip breathing, also known as hypoxic swimming)

50 meters CSS at goal pace to catch breath

500 meters cool-down

Run or ruck 3 miles

#89
MOBILITY DAY

Add in a mobility day when needed; for example, once a week take a full 30–45 minutes devoted to stretching and moving through a full range of motion. On other days, always get a stretch routine in for at least 10–15 minutes. Make stretching an everyday habit like brushing your teeth!

Here is what we do on mobility day:

Warm up for 10–15 minutes with some form of non-impact cardio like bike, elliptical, rower, or swim. Then do a series of dynamic stretches such as Butt-Kickers, Leg Swings (front and

[Continued on next page]

back), Leg Swings (side to side), Side Steps with Lunges, Deep Squat Stretches, or Deep Lunge Stretches. Continue in the pool if available. Treat water with no hands for 10–15 minutes using a variety of kicks such as breast stroke kick, flutterkicks, scissor kicks, or egg beater. Tread water using only your arms for 5 minutes, going back and forth creating lift by angling your hand about 45 degrees when going forward and backward. Then do all the normal dynamic stretches you do on land, but in chest deep water.

#90
NON-IMPACT DAY

Non-impact cardio workout options:

Swim Workout

500 meters, 400 meters, 300 meters, 200 meters, 100 meters

Rest as needed in between sets; focus on goal pace

Bike Workout

Pyramid: Each minute, make resistance higher by two levels for 15 minutes, then repeat in reverse order

Elliptical

Same pyramid as above

[Continued on next page]

Rowing

2000 meters row for time

Add in a Tabata interval: 20 seconds sprint/10 seconds easy for 5 minutes for each of the non-impact options (bike, elliptical, row). If you opt for the swim interval, try 50 meters sprint/25 meters easy for 5 minutes of your swim.

Select 2–3 methods of cardio

#91
CARDIO DAY (WITH OPTIONS)

Long run or ruck day

Run or ruck with 40 pounds as long as you can for 50 minutes. Mix in non-impact exercises (fast bike, elliptical or rowing machine for 2 minutes each set) if this is too much running for you at this time.

Swim with fins 2000 meters

#92
SWIM INTERVAL WORKOUT

500 meters warm-up, any stroke/
   stretch

Swim Workout

Swim 5 x 100 meter sprints

2 x 200 meters at goal swim pace

3 x 100 meter sprints

1 x 200 meter easy

1 x 100 meter sprint

   = 1500 meters swim workout

#93
SWIM OR RUN PT

Swim or Run 30 minutes

Every 5 minutes, stop and do:

Max Push-Ups – 1 minute

Flutterkicks – 1 minute

Plank Pose – 1 minute

#94
SWIM WORKOUT

500 meters warm-up without fins

1000 meters with fins

5 x 100 meters CSS at goal pace
(shoot for 50 second 50 meters
swims = 8:20 500 meters test
score)

10 x 50 meters CSS at goal pace
(shoot for 50 second 50 meters
swims)

Rest as needed in between sets of
100 meters and 50 meters

#95
30 MINUTE SETS OF SPEC OPS TRIATHLON

30 minutes run

30 minutes ruck

30 minutes swim with fins

How far do you get with each event?

#96
SWIM WORKOUT FREESTYLE WITH COMBAT SWIMMER STROKE

Swim Workout

Any stroke 500 meters warm-up/ stretch

Repeat 5 times

50 meters CSS at goal pace

50 meters of 8 strokes per breath hypoxic freestyle

Repeat 5 times

100 meters CSS at goal pace

100 meters of 8 strokes per breath hypoxic freestyle

#97
RUN OR SWIM PT PLUS LONGER COOL-DOWN

Warm up 10 minutes run, swim, bike to warm-up legs

Light stretch

Run or Swim PT

100 meters sprint x 5

After fifth set, do a set of Push-Ups, Sit-Ups – 2 minutes each

200 meters sprint x 4

After fourth set, do Push-Ups, Sit-Ups – 1 minute each

100 meters sprint x 3

[Continued on next page]

After third set, do Burpees – 25 reps (if running) OR do Dive Bomber Push-Ups – 20 or 2 minutes Plank Pose if swimming

200 meters sprint x 1

Abs of choice – 100

100 meters sprint x 1

Cool-down 2–3 miles run or 1500 meters swim with fins

#98
TRACK WORKOUT CHALLENGE

Run 400 meters (see workout below); shoot for the following times each set:

Set 1: 1:40

Set 2: 1:30

Set 3: 1:20

Set 4: 1:10

Set 5: 1:00

Set 6: 1:10

Set 7: 1:20

Set 8: 1:30

Set 9: ¼ mile walking lunges (non-stop)

[Continued on next page]

Rest 1 minute between each set and do your best to hit the time (though some will be tough to get).

Pull-Ups

Max reps x 5 sets

Rest with 50 abs of choice

Swim Workout

Repeat 3 times

500 yards timed

Push-Ups – 2 minutes

Sit-Ups – 2 minutes

#99
RUN AND SWIM WORKOUT

3 miles run

1500 meters Swim

500 meters warm-up any stroke

500 meters with fins

250 meters over/unders with fins:
Swim underwater 25 meters
(kick only) then easy side or
back stroke 25 meters for five
sets, to total 250 meters

Lifesaving Buddy Drag 5 x 25 meters:
switch partners at 25 meters
mark (with fins); if no buddy is
available, tread with no hands
and add an extra 5 minutes

Tread water no hands 5 minutes
(no fins)

#100
SWIM WORKOUT AND RESTING WITH SKILLS

Warm up 500 meters without fins timed (free or CSS)

Tread water 5 minutes without fins (no hands)

1000 meters with fins timed (CSS or freestyle)

Tread water 10 minutes (hold brick, weight, etc. 15–20 pounds) with fins

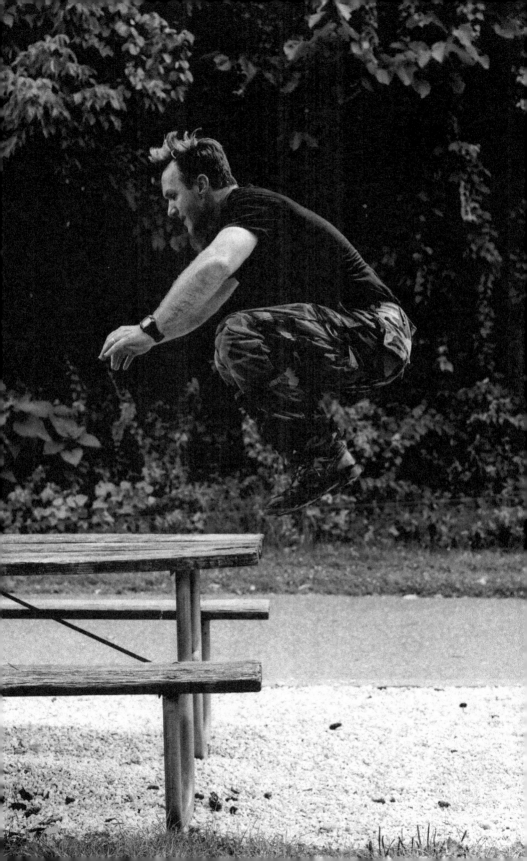

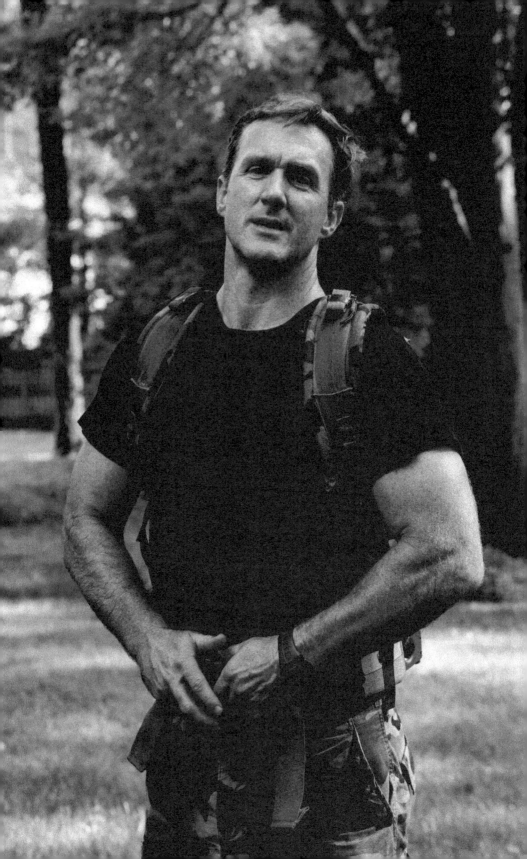

ABOUT THE AUTHOR

Stew Smith, CSCS, is a professional fitness writer with over 20 years of experience in the special ops, military, law enforcement, and firefighting fitness genre, also known as "tactical fitness."

Stew Smith develops fitness training routines that mimic job-related events a tactical operator will need to be successful in training and when operational. Drawing from his Navy SEAL experiences and life-long education and experiences in athletics, preparation for training, as well as coaching others, Stew Smith has developed programs that not only physically prepare you for the tactical life, but also prepare you to deal with everyday issues that require strength, speed, agility, muscle stamina, cardiovascular endurance, and mobility.

He is certified by the National Strength and Conditioning Association as a strength and conditioning specialist (CSCS). His books and downloadable manuals can take you from beginner to a special ops level conditioned tactical athlete. Let these workouts assist you in becoming a better conditioned athlete.

Stew Smith resides near Annapolis, Maryland, where he is actively involved with training tactical athletes who seek special operations, military, police, SWAT, and firefighting professions.

TAKE IT TO THE NEXT LEVEL WITH THESE
MUST-HAVE WORKOUT PROGRAMS

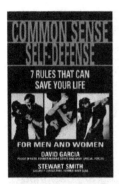

Common Sense Self-Defense

978-1-57826-090-4

*Hand-to-hand combat skills, Spec Ops style!
An essential guide to effective releases and counter
measures designed to defend you against attack.
Protect yourself and your family!*

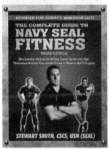

The Complete Guide to Navy Seal
Fitness, Third Edition

978-1-57826-266-3
eBook: 978-1-57826-648-7

*The classic workout program to get you to BUD/S
and beyond, from Navy SEAL legend Stewart Smith.*

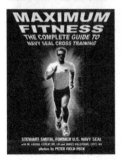

Maximum Fitness

978-1-57826-060-7

*52 weeks of workouts based on scientific period-
ization principles. Train year-round, always gaining.
Strength, cardio and endurance built in.*

Available where books are sold
Also available at www.getfitnow.com

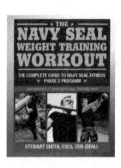
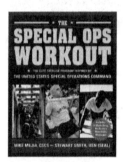
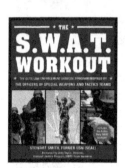

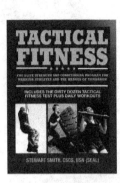

Tactical Fitness

978-1-57826-520-6
eBook: 978-1-57826-521-3
Comprehensive workouts for the warriors of today and the heroes of tomorrow. Includes everything you need to get to it, get through it, and stay with it. Ideal for tactical professionals.

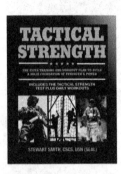

Tactical Strength

978-1-57826-662-3
eBook: 978-1-57826-726-2
Enhance your fitness with an effective strength program built for tactical warriors. Body weight, barbell, dumbbell and odd-object routines challenge you like no other workout!

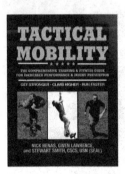

Tactical Mobility

978-1-57826-668-5
eBook: 978-1-57826-669-2
Everyone needs rest and recovery. This program defines optimal programming for improved performance and injury prevention and provides ideal mobility flows to add to your intense training routines and rest days.

Available where books are sold
Also available at www.getfitnow.com

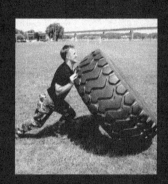 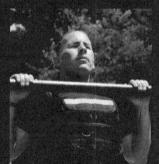 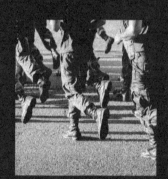

PERSONAL RECORDS

PERSONAL RECORDS

PERSONAL RECORDS

PERSONAL RECORDS